IMG Friendly Emergency Medicine Residency Programs List

With Comprehensive Match Selection Criteria and Programs Requirements

By

IMG Guide

And

Applicant Guide

I0476612

Introduction

Emergency Medicine IMG Friendly Residency Programs List

In Collaboration between the Applicant Guide and the IMG Guide we present to you the most complete and up-to-date IMG friendly Emergency Medicine residency programs list with full match selection criteria and requirements for these programs. This book is essentially written for international medical graduates seeking residency in the US. The idea of writing this book came from our insight that many IMGs every year don't match because they don't know where to apply. Most of the time, they end applying to programs that don't have IMGs or those that don't match their criteria hence they end losing money with no interviews earned. The information was gathered from program directors, coordinators, chiefs, faculty and residents. It includes Programs names, Programs codes, States, Addresses, Phones, Faxes, Percentage of IMGs in the programs, Minimum USMLE Step 1 and Step 2 Score Requirements, Attempts on any step, CS requirement at time of application, USCE Requirements, Cut-Off time since graduation, Programs offering couple match and Visas Sponsored or accepted.

Disclaimer: We are not affiliated to any official or non official organization. We are not affiliated to ECFMG, ERAS, NRMP or USMLE.

Disclaimer: The information in this book is personally collected by the author from various resources in the residency programs which is/are subject to change by/at the programs at any time. Although we did our best to get the most accurate information as much as possible from the program directors, coordinators, faculty and residents, however, you understand that by reading this book you are using the information here on your own responsibility.

Arizona

University of Arizona Emergency Medicine Residency Program

Specialty: Emergency Medicine
Program name: University of Arizona Program
Program code: 110-03-12-056
NRMP Code: 1015110C0
Program type: University-based
State: Arizona
Address: University of Arizona Health Sciences Center, PO Box 245057,
          1501 N Campbell Ave, Tucson, AZ 85724
Phone: (520) 626-7233
Fax: (520) 626-1633

Percentage of IMGs in the program: 10%
Minimum USMLE Step 1 Score Requirement: 220
Minimum USMLE Step 2 Score Requirement: 220
Attempts on any step: Maximum of 2 attempts allowed on each step
CS required at time of application: No
USCE Requirement: None
Cut-Off time since graduation: No limits set
Program offers couple match: Yes
Visas Sponsored or accepted: J1 visa

California

Kaiser Permanente Southern California Emergency Medicine Residency Program

Specialty: Emergency Medicine
Program name: Kaiser Permanente Southern California Program
Program code: 110-05-00-21
State: California
Address: Kaiser Permanente Southern

California, Emergency Medicine Program,
                4647 Zion Ave, San Diego, CA 92120
Phone: (619) 528-5164
Fax: (619) 528-7965
Percentage of IMGs in the program: New program
Minimum USMLE Step 1 Score Requirement: 220
Minimum USMLE Step 2 Score Requirement: 220
Attempts on any step: No limits set
CS required at time of application: Yes as will as ECFMG certificate and PTAL/ Status letter
USCE Requirement: None
Cut-Off time since graduation: No limits set
Program offers couple match: Yes
Visas Sponsored or accepted: No visa

Kern Medical Center Emergency Medicine Residency Program

Specialty: Emergency Medicine
Program name: Kern Medical Center Program
Program code: 110-05-12-001
NRMP Code: 1921110C0
Program type: Community-based university affiliated hospital
State: California
Address: Kern Medical Center, Department of Emergency Medicine,

1700 Mount Vernon Ave, Bakersfield, CA 93306
Phone: (661) 326-2168
Fax: (661) 326-2165
Percentage of IMGs in the program: 10%
Minimum USMLE Step 1 Score Requirement: No limits set
Minimum USMLE Step 2 Score Requirement: No limits set
Attempts on any step: Must pass on first attempt including CS exam
CS required at time of application: No but PTAL/Status letter required
USCE Requirement: None
Cut-Off time since graduation: No limits set
Program offers couple match: Yes
Visas Sponsored or accepted: No visa

Kaweah Delta Health Care District (KDHCD) Emergency Medicine Residency Program

Specialty: Emergency Medicine
Program name: Kaweah Delta Health Care District (KDHCD) Program
Program code: 110-05-00-213
State: California
Address: Kaweah Delta Health Care District, Emergency Medicine Program,
400 W Mineral King Ave, Visalia, CA

93291
Phone: (559) 624-5218
Fax: (559) 741-4845
Percentage of IMGs in the program: 18%
Minimum USMLE Step 1 Score Requirement:
No limits set
Minimum USMLE Step 2 Score Requirement:
No limits set
Attempts on any step: Maximum of 2 attempts
on each step including CS exam
CS required at time of application: Yes
including ECFMG certificate and PTAL/Status
letter
USCE Requirement: None
Cut-Off time since graduation: 3 years
Program offers couple match: Yes
Visas Sponsored or accepted: J1 visa

Connecticut

Yale-New Haven Medical Center Emergency Medicine Residency Program

Specialty: Emergency Medicine

Program name: Yale-New Haven Medical Center Program
Program code: 110-08-21-139
NRMP Code: 1089110C0
Program type: University-based
State: Connecticut
Address: Yale-New Haven Medical Center, Department of Emergency Medicine Suite 260, 464 Congress Ave, New Haven, CT 06519-1315
Phone: (203) 785-5174
Fax: (203) 785-4580
Percentage of IMGs in the program: 8%
Minimum USMLE Step 1 Score Requirement: No limits set
Minimum USMLE Step 2 Score Requirement: No limits set
Attempts on any step: No limits set
CS required at time of application: No
USCE Requirement: None
Cut-Off time since graduation: No limits set
Program offers couple match: Yes
Visas Sponsored or accepted: J1 visa

University of Connecticut Emergency Medicine Residency Program

Specialty: Emergency Medicine

Program name: University of Connecticut Program
Program code: 110-08-21-120
NRMP Code: 1094110C0
Program type: Community-based university affiliated hospital
State: Connecticut
Address: University of Connecticut Health Center, Emergency Medicine Program MC-1930, 263 Farmington Ave, Farmington, CT 06030-1930
Phone: (860) 679-4988
Fax: (860) 679-3489
Percentage of IMGs in the program: 10%
Minimum USMLE Step 1 Score Requirement: 210
Minimum USMLE Step 2 Score Requirement: 210
Attempts on any step: Must pass on first attempt including CS exam
CS required at time of application: No
USCE Requirement: Yes 1 month in any US EM Department
Cut-Off time since graduation: 5 years
Program offers couple match: Yes
Visas Sponsored or accepted: J1 visa

District of Columbia

George Washington University Emergency Medicine Residency Program

Specialty: Emergency Medicine
Program name: George Washington University Program
Program code: 110-10-12-011
NRMP Code: 1802110C0
Program type: University-based
State: District of Columbia
Address: George Washington University Medical Center,
            Department of Emergency Medicine Suite 450,
            2120 L St NW, Washington, DC 20037
Phone: (202) 741-2914
Fax: (202) 741-2921
Percentage of IMGs in the program: 15%
Minimum USMLE Step 1 Score Requirement: No limits set
Minimum USMLE Step 2 Score Requirement: No limits set
Attempts on any step: Two maximum attempts on each step
CS required at time of application: Yes including ECFMG certificate
USCE Requirement: Yes
Cut-Off time since graduation: No limits set
Program offers couple match: Yes
Visas Sponsored or accepted: J1 visa

Florida

University of South Florida Morsani Emergency Medicine Residency Program

Specialty: Emergency Medicine
Program name: University of South Florida Morsani Program
Program code: 110-11-21-167
State: Florida
Address: University of South Florida, Suite 504, One Davis Blvd, Tampa, FL 33606
Phone: (813) 627-5931
Fax: (813) 254-6440
Percentage of IMGs in the program: 10%
Minimum USMLE Step 1 Score Requirement: No limits set
Minimum USMLE Step 2 Score Requirement: No limits set
Attempts on any step: No limits set
CS required at time of application: No
USCE Requirement: None
Cut-Off time since graduation: No limits set
Program offers couple match: Yes
Visas Sponsored or accepted: J1 visa

Orlando Health Emergency Medicine Residency Program

Specialty: Emergency Medicine
Program name: Orlando Health Program
Program code: 110-11-21-072
NRMP Code: 1107110C0
Program type: Community-based university affiliated hospital
State: Florida
Address: Orlando Regional Medical Center,
Department of Emergency Medicine Suite 200,
86 W Underwood St, Orlando, FL 32806-2134
Phone: (407) 237-6329
Fax: (407) 649-3083
Percentage of IMGs in the program: 5%
Minimum USMLE Step 1 Score Requirement: 210
Minimum USMLE Step 2 Score Requirement: 210
Attempts on any step: Must pass on first attempt including CS exam
CS required at time of application: No
USCE Requirement: None
Cut-Off time since graduation: 3 years
Program offers couple match: Yes
Visas Sponsored or accepted: J1 visa

Florida Hospital Medical Center Emergency Medicine Residency Program

Specialty: Emergency Medicine
Program name: Florida Hospital Medical Center Program
Program code: 110-11-12-190
NRMP Code: 1102110C0
Program type: Community-based university affiliated hospital
State: Florida
Address: Florida Hospital, Emergency Medicine Program,
          7727 Lake Underhill Rd, Orlando, FL 32822
Phone: (407) 303-6413
Fax: (407) 303-6414
Percentage of IMGs in the program: 10%
Minimum USMLE Step 1 Score Requirement: No limits set
Minimum USMLE Step 2 Score Requirement: No limits set
Attempts on any step: No limits set
CS required at time of application: No
USCE Requirement: None
Cut-Off time since graduation: No limits set
Program offers couple match: Yes
Visas Sponsored or accepted: J1 visa and H1b visa

University of Florida Emergency Medicine Residency Program

Specialty: Emergency Medicine
Program name: University of Florida Program
Program code: 110-11-31-186
NRMP Code: 1824110C0
Program type: University-based
State: Florida
Address: University of Florida College of Medicine,

Department of Emergency Medicine Rm 4270,

1329 SW 16th St, Gainesville, FL 32610,

Phone: (352) 265-5911
Fax: (352) 265-5606
Percentage of IMGs in the program: 5%
Minimum USMLE Step 1 Score Requirement: No limits set
Minimum USMLE Step 2 Score Requirement: No limits set
Attempts on any step: No limits set
CS required at time of application: Yes
USCE Requirement: Yes
Cut-Off time since graduation: No limits set
Program offers couple match: Yes
Visas Sponsored or accepted: No visa

Georgia

Medical College of Georgia Emergency Medicine Residency Program

Specialty: Emergency Medicine
Program name: Medical College of Georgia Program
Program code: 110-12-21-090
NRMP Code: 1985110C0
Program type: University-based
State: Georgia
Address: Georgia Regents University MCG
1120 15th St, Augusta, GA 30912-2800
Phone: (706) 721-2613
Fax: (706) 721-9081
Percentage of IMGs in the program: 5%
Minimum USMLE Step 1 Score Requirement: No limits set
Minimum USMLE Step 2 Score Requirement: No limits set
Attempts on any step: No limits set
CS required at time of application: No
USCE Requirement: None
Cut-Off time since graduation: No limits set
Program offers couple match: Yes
Visas Sponsored or accepted: J1 visa

Emory University Emergency Medicine Residency Program

Specialty: Emergency Medicine
Program name: Emory University Program
Program code: 110-12-12-012
NRMP Code: 1113110C0, 1113110C1
Program type: University-based
State: Georgia
Address: Grady Memorial Hospital
49 Jesse Hill Jr Dr SE, Atlanta, GA 30303-3219
Phone: (404) 251-8865
Fax: (404) 688-6355
Percentage of IMGs in the program: 10%
Minimum USMLE Step 1 Score Requirement: No limits set
Minimum USMLE Step 2 Score Requirement: No limits set
Attempts on any step: Must pass from maximum the 2nd attempt on any step including CS exam
CS required at time of application: No
USCE Requirement: None
Cut-Off time since graduation: No limits set
Program offers couple match: Yes
Visas Sponsored or accepted: H1b visa

Illinois

Presence Resurrection Medical Center Emergency Medicine Residency Program

Specialty: Emergency Medicine
Program name: Presence Resurrection Medical Center Program
Program code: 110-16-31-146
NRMP Code: 1937110C0
Program type: Community-based
State: Illinois
Address: Presence Resurrection Medical Center
7435 W Talcott Ave, Chicago, IL 60631-3746
Phone: (773) 990-6550
Fax: (773) 594-7805
Percentage of IMGs in the program: 4%
Minimum USMLE Step 1 Score Requirement: No limits set
Minimum USMLE Step 2 Score Requirement: No limits set
Attempts on any step: No limits set
CS required at time of application: No
USCE Requirement: None
Cut-Off time since graduation: No limits set
Program offers couple match: Yes
Visas Sponsored or accepted: No visa

John H Stroger Hospital of Cook County Emergency Medicine Residency Program

Specialty: Emergency Medicine
Program name: John H Stroger Hospital of Cook County Program
Program code: 110-16-21-083
State: Illinois
Address: Stroger Hospital of Cook County
1900 W Polk St, Chicago, IL 60612
Phone: (312) 864-0062
Fax: (312) 864-9656
Percentage of IMGs in the program: 5%
Minimum USMLE Step 1 Score Requirement: No limits set
Minimum USMLE Step 2 Score Requirement: No limits set
Attempts on any step: Must pass on first attempt
CS required at time of application: No
USCE Requirement: Yes
Cut-Off time since graduation: No limits set
Program offers couple match: Yes
Visas Sponsored or accepted: J1 visa and H1b visa

Louisiana

Louisiana State University (Shreveport) Emergency Medicine Residency Program

Specialty: Emergency Medicine
Program name: Louisiana State University (Shreveport) Program
Program code: 110-21-22-170
State: Louisiana
Address: LSU Health Science Center Shreveport
1541 Kings Highway, Shreveport, LA 71130-3932
Phone: (318) 675-6632
Fax: (318) 675-6878
Percentage of IMGs in the program: 20%
Minimum USMLE Step 1 Score Requirement: 220
Minimum USMLE Step 2 Score Requirement: 220
Attempts on any step: Must pass on maximum 2nd attempt on each step including CS exam
CS required at time of application: No
USCE Requirement: None
Cut-Off time since graduation: No limits set
Program offers couple match: Yes
Visas Sponsored or accepted: J1 visa

Earl K Long Medical Center/Louisiana State University (Baton Rouge) Emergency Medicine Residency Program

Specialty: Emergency Medicine
Program name: Earl K Long Medical Center/Louisiana State University (Baton Rouge) Program
Program code: 110-21-21-117
State: Louisiana
Address: LSU Baton Rouge
          7556 Hennessy Blvd, Baton Rouge, LA 70808
Phone: (225) 374-0046
Fax: (225) 765-0961
Percentage of IMGs in the program: 15%
Minimum USMLE Step 1 Score Requirement: No limits set
Minimum USMLE Step 2 Score Requirement: No limits set
Attempts on any step: Must pass on maximum 2nd attempt on each step including CS exam
CS required at time of application: Yes including ECFMG certificate
USCE Requirement: None
Cut-Off time since graduation: No limits set
Program offers couple match: Yes
Visas Sponsored or accepted: J1 visa

Maryland

University of Maryland Emergency Medicine Residency Program

Specialty: Emergency Medicine
Program name: University of Maryland Program
Program code: 110-23-21-101
NRMP Code: 1252110C0
Program type: University-based
State: Maryland
Address: University of Maryland Medical System

      110 S Paca St, Baltimore, MD 21201
Phone: (410) 328-9702
Fax: (410) 328-8028
Percentage of IMGs in the program: 10%
Minimum USMLE Step 1 Score Requirement: No limits set
Minimum USMLE Step 2 Score Requirement: No limits set
Attempts on any step: No limits set
CS required at time of application: Yes including ECFMG certificate
USCE Requirement: None, but preference given to those who did Transitional/Prelim year
Cut-Off time since graduation: No limits set

Program offers couple match: Yes
Visas Sponsored or accepted: No visa

Johns Hopkins University Emergency Medicine Residency Program

Specialty: Emergency Medicine
Program name: Johns Hopkins University Program
Program code: 110-23-12-022
State: Maryland
Address: Johns Hopkins University Hospital
1830 E Monument St, Baltimore, MD 21287-2080
Phone: (410) 955-5107
Fax: (410) 502-5146
Percentage of IMGs in the program: 0% (Occasionally one)
Minimum USMLE Step 1 Score Requirement: No limits set
Minimum USMLE Step 2 Score Requirement: No limits set
Attempts on any step: Must pass on first attempt including CS exam
CS required at time of application: Yes including ECFMG certificate
USCE Requirement: Yes, 1 year
Cut-Off time since graduation: 2 years
Program offers couple match: Yes

Visas Sponsored or accepted: J1 visa

Massachusetts

Baystate Medical Center/Tufts University School of Medicine Emergency Medicine Residency Program

Specialty: Emergency Medicine
Program name: Baystate Medical Center/Tufts University School of Medicine Program
Program code: 110-24-21-116
NRMP Code: 1286110C0
Program type: Community-based university affiliated hospital
State: Massachusetts
Address: Baystate Medical Center
759 Chestnut St, Springfield, MA 01199
Phone: (413) 794-5999
Fax: (413) 794-8070
Percentage of IMGs in the program: 15%
Minimum USMLE Step 1 Score Requirement: No limits set

Minimum USMLE Step 2 Score
Requirement: No limits set
Attempts on any step: Must pass from
maximum the 2nd attempt on each step
CS required at time of application: No
USCE Requirement: None
Cut-Off time since graduation: No limits set
Program offers couple match: Yes
Visas Sponsored or accepted: J1 visa

Boston Medical Center Emergency Medicine Residency Program

Specialty: Emergency Medicine
Program name: Boston Medical Center Program
Program code: 110-24-21-084
NRMP Code: 1257110C0
Program type: University-based
State: Massachusetts
Address: Boston University Medical Center
           One Boston Medical Center Pl, Boston,
MA 02118
Phone: (617) 414-4929
Fax: (617) 414-7759
Percentage of IMGs in the program: 5%
Minimum USMLE Step 1 Score Requirement:
No limits set
Minimum USMLE Step 2 Score
Requirement: No limits set

Attempts on any step: No limits set
CS required at time of application: Yes including ECFMG certificate
USCE Requirement: None
Cut-Off time since graduation: No limits set
Program offers couple match: Yes
Visas Sponsored or accepted: J1 visa

University of Massachusetts Emergency Medicine Residency Program

Specialty: Emergency Medicine
Program name: University of Massachusetts Program
Program code: 110-24-21-074
NRMP Code: 3050110C0
Program type: University-based
State: Massachusetts
Address: University of Massachusetts Medical School
        55 Lake Ave N, Worcester, MA 01655
Phone: (508) 421-1439
Fax: (508) 421-1490
Percentage of IMGs in the program:
5% variable
Minimum USMLE Step 1 Score Requirement:
210
Minimum USMLE Step 2 Score Requirement:
210

Attempts on any step: No limits set
CS required at time of application: No
USCE Requirement: None
Cut-Off time since graduation: No limits set
Program offers couple match: Yes
Visas Sponsored or accepted: J1 visa

Michigan

St John Hospital and Medical Center Emergency Medicine Residency Program

Specialty: Emergency Medicine
Program name: St John Hospital and Medical Center Program
Program code: 110-25-21-132
NRMP Code: 1915110C0
Program type: Community-based university affiliated hospital
State: Michigan
Address: St John Hospital and Medical Center
19251 Mack Ave, Grosse Pointe Woods, MI 48236
Phone: (313) 343-3875
Fax: (313) 343-7840
Percentage of IMGs in the program: 5%
Minimum USMLE Step 1 Score Requirement: No limits set

Minimum USMLE Step 2 Score Requirement:
No limits set
Attempts on any step: Must pass on first attempt
CS required at time of application: No
USCE Requirement: None
Cut-Off time since graduation: 3 years
Program offers couple match: Yes
Visas Sponsored or accepted: J1 visa and H1b visa

Western Michigan University School of Medicine Emergency Medicine Residency Program

Specialty: Emergency Medicine
Program name: Western Michigan University School of Medicine Program
Program code: 110-25-21-124
NRMP Code: 1314110C0
Program type: Community-based University affiliated hospital
State: Michigan
Address: Western Michigan University School of Medicine
          1000 Oakland Dr, Kalamazoo, MI 49008-8060
Phone: (269) 337-6600
Fax: (269) 337-6475
Percentage of IMGs in the program: 5%

Minimum USMLE Step 1 Score Requirement:
No limits set
Minimum USMLE Step 2 Score Requirement:
No limits set
Attempts on any step: Must pass on first attempt
CS required at time of application: No
USCE Requirement: None
Cut-Off time since graduation: 5 years
Program offers couple match: Yes
Visas Sponsored or accepted: No visa

Genesys Regional Medical Center Emergency Medicine Residency Program

Specialty: Emergency Medicine
Program name: Genesys Regional Medical Center Program
Program code: 110-25-13-196
State: Michigan
Address: Genesys Regional Medical Center
One Genesys Pkwy, Grand Blanc, MI 48439
Phone: (810) 606-6372
Fax: (810) 606-5990
Percentage of IMGs in the program: 20%
Minimum USMLE Step 1 Score Requirement:
215

Minimum USMLE Step 2 Score Requirement: 215
Attempts on any step: Must pass on first attempt on any step including CS exam
CS required at time of application: No
USCE Requirement: None
Cut-Off time since graduation: 3 years
Program offers couple match: Yes
Visas Sponsored or accepted: No visa

Sparrow Hospital/Michigan State University Emergency Medicine Residency Program

Specialty: Emergency Medicine
Program name: Sparrow Hospital/Michigan State University Program
Program code: 110-25-12-027
NRMP Code: 1315110C0
Program type: Community-based university affiliated hospital
State: Michigan
Address: Sparrow Hospital
          1215 E Michigan Ave, Lansing, MI 48909
Phone: (517) 364-2583
Fax: (517) 364-3002

Percentage of IMGs in the program: 0% (occasionally one)
Minimum USMLE Step 1 Score Requirement: No limits set
Minimum USMLE Step 2 Score Requirement: No limits set
Attempts on any step: Must pass on first attempt including CS exam
CS required at time of application: Yes including ECFMG certificate
USCE Requirement: None
Cut-Off time since graduation: No limits set
Program offers couple match: Yes
Visas Sponsored or accepted: J1 visa

Henry Ford Hospital/Wayne State University Emergency Medicine Residency Program

Specialty: Emergency Medicine
Program name: Henry Ford Hospital/Wayne State University Program
Program code: 110-25-12-025
NRMP Code: 1300110C0
Program type: Community-based university affiliated hospital
State: Michigan
Address: Henry Ford Hospital
2799 W Grand Blvd, Detroit, MI 48202

Phone: (313) 916-1553
Fax: (313) 916-7437
Percentage of IMGs in the program: 8%
Minimum USMLE Step 1 Score Requirement: No limits set
Minimum USMLE Step 2 Score Requirement: No limits set
Attempts on any step: No limits set
CS required at time of application: Yes
USCE Requirement: None
Cut-Off time since graduation: No limits set
Program offers couple match: Yes
Visas Sponsored or accepted: J1 visa

Central Michigan University College of Medicine Emergency Medicine Residency Program

Specialty: Emergency Medicine
Program name: Central Michigan University College of Medicine Program
Program code: 110-25-11-138
NRMP Code: 1320110C0, 1320110C1
Program type: Community-based university affiliated hospital
State: Michigan
Address: Central Michigan University College of Medicine
1000 Houghton Ave, Saginaw, MI

48602
Phone: (989) 583-6817
Fax: (989) 583-7436
Percentage of IMGs in the program: 20%
Minimum USMLE Step 1 Score Requirement: No limits set
Minimum USMLE Step 2 Score Requirement: No limits set
Attempts on any step: Must pass on first attempt on any step
CS required at time of application: No
USCE Requirement: Yes, 3 months
Cut-Off time since graduation: 2 years
Program offers couple match: Yes
Visas Sponsored or accepted: No visa

Minnesota

Mayo Clinic College of Medicine (Rochester) Emergency Medicine Residency Program

Specialty: Emergency Medicine
Program name: Mayo Clinic College of Medicine (Rochester) Program
Program code: 110-26-21-161

NRMP Code: 1328110C0
Program type: University-based
State: Minnesota
Address: St Marys Hospital
 1216 Second St SW, Rochester, MN 55902
Phone: (507) 255-2192
Fax: (507) 255-6592
Percentage of IMGs in the program: 5%
Minimum USMLE Step 1 Score Requirement: No limits set
Minimum USMLE Step 2 Score Requirement: No limits set
Attempts on any step: No limits set
CS required at time of application: Yes including ECFMG certificate
USCE Requirement: None
Cut-Off time since graduation: No limits set
Program offers couple match: Yes
Visas Sponsored or accepted: J1 visa

Mississippi

University of Mississippi Medical Center Emergency Medicine Residency Program

Specialty: Emergency Medicine
Program name: University of Mississippi Medical Center Program
Program code: 110-27-21-073
NRMP Code: 1957110C0
Program type: University-based
State: Mississippi
Address: University of Mississippi Med Center, Department of Emergency Medicine,
          2500 N State St, Jackson, MS 39216-4505
Phone: (601) 984-5582
Fax: (601) 984-5583
Percentage of IMGs in the program: 18%
Minimum USMLE Step 1 Score Requirement: No limits set
Minimum USMLE Step 2 Score Requirement: No limits set
Attempts on any step: Must pass on first attempt including CS exam
CS required at time of application: No
USCE Requirement: None
Cut-Off time since graduation: No limits set
Program offers couple match: Yes
Visas Sponsored or accepted: J1 visa

New Jersey

Rutgers New Jersey Medical School Emergency Medicine Residency Program

Specialty: Emergency Medicine
Program name: Rutgers New Jersey Medical School Program
Program code: 110-33-31-177
NRMP Code: 1398110C0
Program type: University-based
State: New Jersey
Address: Rutgers New Jersey Medical School
30 Bergen St, Newark, NJ 07103
Phone: (973) 972-9261
Fax: (973) 972-9268
Percentage of IMGs in the program: 10% (Variable)
Minimum USMLE Step 1 Score Requirement: 210
Minimum USMLE Step 2 Score Requirement: 210
Attempts on any step: Must pass on first attempt including CS exam
CS required at time of application: Yes
USCE Requirement: Yes, 12 months
Cut-Off time since graduation: No limits set
Program offers couple match: No
Visas Sponsored or accepted: J1 visa

Rutgers Robert Wood Johnson Medical School Emergency Medicine Residency Program

Specialty: Emergency Medicine
Program name: Rutgers Robert Wood Johnson Medical School Program
Program code: 110-33-21-205
State: New Jersey
Address: Rutgers Robert Wood Johnson Medical School
　　　　　One Robert Wood Johnson Pl, New Brunswick, NJ 08901
Phone: (732) 235-4296
Fax: (732) 235-6434
Percentage of IMGs in the program: 20%
Minimum USMLE Step 1 Score Requirement: No limits set
Minimum USMLE Step 2 Score Requirement: No limits set
Attempts on any step: Must pass on first attempt
CS required at time of application: No
USCE Requirement: None
Cut-Off time since graduation: No limits set
Program offers couple match: Yes
Visas Sponsored or accepted: J1 visa

Newark Beth Israel Medical Center Emergency Medicine Residency Program

Specialty: Emergency Medicine
Program name: Newark Beth Israel Medical Center Program
Program code: 110-33-21-158
NRMP Code: 1397110C0
Program type: Community-based university affiliated hospital
State: New Jersey
Address: Newark Beth Israel Medical Centre
201 Lyons Ave, Newark, NJ 07112
Phone: (973) 926-6671
Fax: (973) 282-0562
Percentage of IMGs in the program: 30%
Minimum USMLE Step 1 Score Requirement: No limits set
Minimum USMLE Step 2 Score Requirement: No limits set
Attempts on any step: Must pass on first attempt including CS exam
CS required at time of application: No
USCE Requirement: None
Cut-Off time since graduation: No limits set
Program offers couple match: No
Visas Sponsored or accepted: J1 visa

Hackensack University Medical Center Emergency Medicine Residency Program

Specialty: Emergency Medicine
Program name: Hackensack University Medical Center Program
Program code: 110-33-00-213
Program type: University-based
State: New Jersey
Address: Hackensack University Medical Center
        30 Prospect Ave, Hackensack, NJ 07601
Phone: (201) 996-3307
Fax: (201) 996-4239
Percentage of IMGs in the program: 25%
Minimum USMLE Step 1 Score Requirement: No limits set
Minimum USMLE Step 2 Score Requirement: No limits set
Attempts on any step: No limits set
CS required at time of application: Yes including ECFMG certificate
USCE Requirement: None
Cut-Off time since graduation: No limits set
Program offers couple match: Yes
Visas Sponsored or accepted: J1 visa

New York Medical College at St Joseph's Regional Medical Center Emergency Medicine Residency Program

Specialty: Emergency Medicine
Program name: New York Medical College at St Joseph's Regional Medical Center Program
Program code: 110-33-00-212
State: New Jersey
Address: St Joseph's Regional Medical Center
703 Main St, Paterson, NJ 07503
Phone: (973) 754-2248
Fax: (973) 754-2516
Percentage of IMGs in the program: 25%
Minimum USMLE Step 1 Score Requirement: No limits set
Minimum USMLE Step 2 Score Requirement: No limits set
Attempts on any step: No limits set
CS required at time of application: Yes including ECFMG certificate
USCE Requirement: None
Cut-Off time since graduation: No limits set
Program offers couple match: Yes
Visas Sponsored or accepted: J1 visa

New Mexico

University of New Mexico Emergency Medicine Residency Program

Specialty: Emergency Medicine
Program name: University of New Mexico Program
Program code: 110-34-21-075
NRMP Code: 1962110C0
Program type: University-based
State: New Mexico
Address: University of New Mexico Health Science Center
1 Univ of New Mexico, Albuquerque, NM 87131-0001
Phone: (505) 272-6524
Fax: (505) 272-6503
Percentage of IMGs in the program: 10%
Minimum USMLE Step 1 Score Requirement: No limits set
Minimum USMLE Step 2 Score Requirement: No limits set
Attempts on any step: No limits set
CS required at time of application: Yes including ECFMG certificate
USCE Requirement: None
Cut-Off time since graduation: No limits set
Program offers couple match: Yes

Visas Sponsored or accepted: J1 visa

New York

SUNY Health Science Center at Brooklyn Emergency Medicine Residency Program

Specialty: Emergency Medicine
Program name: SUNY Health Science Center at Brooklyn Program
Program code: 110-35-31-135
State: New York
Address: SUNY Downstate Medical Center
450 Clarkson Ave, Brooklyn, NY 11203
Phone: (718) 245-3318
Fax: (718) 245-4799
Percentage of IMGs in the program: 0%
(Occasionally 1 from Saudi affiliated Universities)
Minimum USMLE Step 1 Score Requirement: No limits set
Minimum USMLE Step 2 Score Requirement: No limits set
Attempts on any step: No limits set
CS required at time of application: No
USCE Requirement: None

Cut-Off time since graduation: No limits set
Program offers couple match: Yes
Visas Sponsored or accepted: J1 visa and H1b visa

Maimonides Medical Center Emergency Medicine Residency Program

Specialty: Emergency Medicine
Program name: Maimonides Medical Center Program
Program code: 110-35-21-164
NRMP Code: 1428110C0
Program type: Community-based university affiliated hospital
State: New York
Address: Maimonides Medical Center
4802 Tenth Ave, Brooklyn, NY 11219
Phone: (718) 283-6029
Fax: (718) 635-7228
Percentage of IMGs in the program: 15%
Minimum USMLE Step 1 Score Requirement: 205
Minimum USMLE Step 2 Score Requirement: 205
Attempts on any step: Must pass on first attempt
CS required at time of application: No
USCE Requirement: Yes

Cut-Off time since graduation: 5 years
Program offers couple match: No
Visas Sponsored or accepted: J1 visa and H1b visa

New York Methodist Hospital Emergency Medicine Residency Program

Specialty: Emergency Medicine
Program name: New York Methodist Hospital Program
Program code: 110-35-21-147
NRMP Code: 1429110C0
Program type: Community-based university affiliated hospital
State: New York
Address: New York Methodist Hospital
506 Sixth St, Brooklyn, NY 11215
Phone: (718) 780-5042
Fax: (718) 780-3153
Percentage of IMGs in the program: 10%
Minimum USMLE Step 1 Score Requirement: No limits set
Minimum USMLE Step 2 Score Requirement: No limits set
Attempts on any step: No limits set
CS required at time of application: Yes
USCE Requirement: None
Cut-Off time since graduation: No limits set

Program offers couple match: No
Visas Sponsored or accepted: No visa

NSLIJHS/Hofstra North Shore-LIJ School of Medicine at North Shore University Hospital Emergency Medicine Residency Program

Specialty: Emergency Medicine
Program name: NSLIJHS/Hofstra North Shore-LIJ School of Medicine at North Shore University Hospital Program
Program code: 110-35-21-141
NRMP Code: 1700110C0
Program type: University-based
State: New York
Address: North Shore University Hospital
300 Community Dr, Manhasset, NY 11030
Phone: (516) 562-2925
Fax: (516) 562-3569
Percentage of IMGs in the program: 15%
Minimum USMLE Step 1 Score Requirement: No limits set
Minimum USMLE Step 2 Score Requirement: No limits set
Attempts on any step: No limits set
CS required at time of application: Yes
USCE Requirement: None
Cut-Off time since graduation: No limits set

Program offers couple match: No
Visas Sponsored or accepted: J1 visa and H1b visa

SUNY Upstate Medical University Emergency Medicine Residency Program

Specialty: Emergency Medicine
Program name: SUNY Upstate Medical University Program
Program code: 110-35-21-121
NRMP Code: 1516110C0
Program type: University-based
State: New York
Address: SUNY Upstate Medical University
        550 E Genesee St, Syracuse, NY 13202
Phone: (315) 464-4363
Fax: (315) 464-4854
Percentage of IMGs in the program: 20%
Minimum USMLE Step 1 Score Requirement: No limits set
Minimum USMLE Step 2 Score Requirement: No limits set
Attempts on any step: No limits set
CS required at time of application: Yes including ECFMG certificate
USCE Requirement: Yes, 1 month
Cut-Off time since graduation: No limits set

Program offers couple match: Yes
Visas Sponsored or accepted: J1 visa

Brooklyn Hospital Center Emergency Medicine Residency Program

Specialty: Emergency Medicine
Program name: Brooklyn Hospital Center Program
Program code: 110-35-21-093
NRMP Code: 1420110C0
Program type: Community-based university affiliated hospital
State: New York
Address: Brooklyn Hospital Center
            121 DeKalb Ave, Brooklyn, NY 11201
Phone: (718) 250-8369
Fax: (718) 250-6528
Percentage of IMGs in the program: 20%
Minimum USMLE Step 1 Score Requirement: 210
Minimum USMLE Step 2 Score Requirement: 210
Attempts on any step: No limits set
CS required at time of application: No
USCE Requirement: None
Cut-Off time since graduation: No limits set
Program offers couple match: Yes

Visas Sponsored or accepted: J1 visa

Lincoln Medical and Mental Health Center Emergency Medicine Residency Program

Specialty: Emergency Medicine
Program name: Lincoln Medical and Mental Health Center Program
Program code: 110-35-12-053
NRMP Code: 1484110C0
Program type: Community-based university affiliated hospital
State: New York
Address: Lincoln Medical and Mental Health Center

       234 E 149th St, Bronx, NY 10451
Phone: (718) 579-6011
Fax: (718) 579-4822
Percentage of IMGs in the program: 40%
Minimum USMLE Step 1 Score Requirement: 215
Minimum USMLE Step 2 Score Requirement: 215
Attempts on any step: No limits set
CS required at time of application: Yes including ECFMG certificate
USCE Requirement: None
Cut-Off time since graduation: No limits set

Program offers couple match: No
Visas Sponsored or accepted: J1 visa

New York Medical College (Metropolitan) Emergency Medicine Residency Program

Specialty: Emergency Medicine
Program name: New York Medical College (Metropolitan) Program
Program code: 110-35-12-031
State: New York
Address: Metropolitan Hospital Center
1901 First Ave, New York, NY 10029
Phone: (212) 423-6684
Fax: (212) 423-6383
Percentage of IMGs in the program: 35%
Minimum USMLE Step 1 Score Requirement: 220
Minimum USMLE Step 2 Score Requirement: 220
Attempts on any step: No limits set
CS required at time of application: Yes including ECFMG certificate
USCE Requirement: None but advantage given to those done rotation in their department
Cut-Off time since graduation: 3 years
Program offers couple match: Yes
Visas Sponsored or accepted: J1 visa and H1b visa

Albert Einstein College of Medicine (Jacobi/Montefiore) Emergency Medicine Residency Program

Specialty: Emergency Medicine
Program name: Albert Einstein College of Medicine (Jacobi/Montefiore) Program
Program code: 110-35-12-030
NRMP Code: 3172110C0
Program type: University-based
State: New York
Address: Jacobi Medical Center
             1400 Pelham Pkwy S, Bronx, NY 10461
Phone: (718) 918-5820
Fax: (718) 918-7459
Percentage of IMGs in the program: 0% (occasionally one)
Minimum USMLE Step 1 Score Requirement: No limits set
Minimum USMLE Step 2 Score Requirement: No limits set
Attempts on any step: Must pass on first attempt including CS exam
CS required at time of application: No
USCE Requirement: None
Cut-Off time since graduation: 4 years
Program offers couple match: Yes

Visas Sponsored or accepted: J1 visa and H1b visa

North Carolina

Duke University Hospital Emergency Medicine Residency Program

Specialty: Emergency Medicine
Program name: Duke University Hospital Program
Program code: 110-36-13-166
State: North Carolina
Address: Duke University Medical Center
2301 Erwin Road, Duke North, Suite 2600, Durham, NC 27710
Phone: (919) 681-2274
Fax: (919) 668-6115
Percentage of IMGs in the program: 0-5% (Variable)
Minimum USMLE Step 1 Score Requirement: No limits set
Minimum USMLE Step 2 Score Requirement: No limits set
Attempts on any step: No limits set

CS required at time of application: Yes including ECFMG certificate
USCE Requirement: None
Cut-Off time since graduation: No limits set
Program offers couple match: Yes
Visas Sponsored or accepted: J1 visa

Ohio

University of Toledo Emergency Medicine Residency Program

Specialty: Emergency Medicine
Program name: University of Toledo Program
Program code: 110-38-12-198
NRMP Code: 1579110C0
Program type: University-based
State: Ohio
Address: University of Toledo Medical Center
            3045 Arlington Ave, Toledo, OH 43614
Phone: (419) 383-6369
Fax: (419) 383-3357
Percentage of IMGs in the program: 20%
Minimum USMLE Step 1 Score Requirement: 215
Minimum USMLE Step 2 Score Requirement: 215

Attempts on any step: No limits set
CS required at time of application: Yes
including ECFMG certificate
USCE Requirement: None
Cut-Off time since graduation: 5 years
Program offers couple match: Yes
Visas Sponsored or accepted: No visa

Mercy St Vincent Medical Center/Mercy Health Partners Emergency Medicine Residency Program

Specialty: Emergency Medicine
Program name: Mercy St Vincent Medical
Center/Mercy Health Partners Program
Program code: 110-38-12-040
State: Ohio
Address: Mercy St Vincent Medical Center
2213 Cherry St, Toledo, OH 43608
Phone: (419) 251-4724
Fax: (419) 251-2698
Percentage of IMGs in the program: 10%
Minimum USMLE Step 1 Score Requirement:
No limits set
Minimum USMLE Step 2 Score Requirement:
No limits set
Attempts on any step: Must pass on first
attempt including CS exam

CS required at time of application: Yes including ECFMG certificate
USCE Requirement: Yes
Cut-Off time since graduation: 5 years
Program offers couple match: Yes
Visas Sponsored or accepted: J1 visa (and H1b visa for exceptional candidates)

Akron General Medical Center/NEOMED Emergency Medicine Residency Program

Specialty: Emergency Medicine
Program name: Akron General Medical Center/NEOMED Program
Program code: 110-38-12-035
State: Ohio
Address: Akron General Medical Center
400 Wabash Ave, Akron, OH 44307
Phone: (330) 344-6326
Fax: (330) 253-8293
Percentage of IMGs in the program: 0-5% (variable)
Minimum USMLE Step 1 Score Requirement: 220
Minimum USMLE Step 2 Score Requirement: 220
Attempts on any step: Must pass on first attempt
CS required at time of application: No

USCE Requirement: None
Cut-Off time since graduation: 5 years
Program offers couple match: Yes
Visas Sponsored or accepted: J1 visa and H1b visa

Summa Health System/NEOMED Emergency Medicine Residency Program

Specialty: Emergency Medicine
Program name: Summa Health System/NEOMED Program
Program code: 110-38-12-034
NRMP Code: 1541110C0
Program type: Community-based university affiliated hospital
State: Ohio
Address: Summa Akron City Hospital
525 E Market St, Akron, OH 44309
Phone: (330) 375-4021
Fax: (330) 375-7564
Percentage of IMGs in the program: 15%
Minimum USMLE Step 1 Score Requirement: No limits set
Minimum USMLE Step 2 Score Requirement: No limits set
Attempts on any step: No limits set
CS required at time of application: Yes
USCE Requirement: None

Cut-Off time since graduation: 4 years
Program offers couple match: Yes
Visas Sponsored or accepted: J1 visa

Pennsylvania

Penn State Milton S Hershey Medical Center Emergency Medicine Residency Program

Specialty: Emergency Medicine
Program name: Penn State Milton S Hershey
Medical Center Program
Program code: 110-41-33-171
NRMP Code: 1617110C0
Program type: University-based
State: Pennsylvania
Address: Penn State Hershey Medical Center
500 University Dr, Hershey, PA 17033
Phone: (717) 531-1443
Fax: (717) 531-4441
Percentage of IMGs in the program: 10%
Minimum USMLE Step 1 Score Requirement:
No limits set

Minimum USMLE Step 2 Score Requirement:
No limits set
Attempts on any step: Must pass on first attempt
CS required at time of application: No
USCE Requirement: None
Cut-Off time since graduation: 5 years
Program offers couple match: Yes
Visas Sponsored or accepted: J1 visa

Lehigh Valley Health Network/University of South Florida College of Medicine Emergency Medicine Residency Program

Specialty: Emergency Medicine
Program name: Lehigh Valley Health Network/University of South Florida College of Medicine Program
Program code: 110-41-21-199
NRMP Code: 1601110C0
Program type: Community-based university affiliated hospital
State: Pennsylvania
Address: Lehigh Valley Hosp (Muhlenberg)
2545 Schoenersville Rd, Bethlehem, PA 18017
Phone: (484) 884-2888

Fax: (484) 884-2885
Percentage of IMGs in the program: 5%
Minimum USMLE Step 1 Score Requirement: No limits set
Minimum USMLE Step 2 Score Requirement: No limits set
Attempts on any step: Must pass on first attempt including CS exam
CS required at time of application: Yes
USCE Requirement: None
Cut-Off time since graduation: No limits set
Program offers couple match: Yes
Visas Sponsored or accepted: J1 visa

University of Pennsylvania Emergency Medicine Residency Program

Specialty: Emergency Medicine
Program name: University of Pennsylvania Program
Program code: 110-41-21-148
State: Pennsylvania
Address: Hospital of University of Pennsylvania Dept of Emergency Med Ground Ravdin
3400 Spruce St
Philadelphia, PA 19104
Phone: (215) 662-6305
Fax: (215) 662-2875

Percentage of IMGs in the program: 0% (occasionally one)
Minimum USMLE Step 1 Score Requirement: No limits set
Minimum USMLE Step 2 Score Requirement: No limits set
Attempts on any step: No limits set
CS required at time of application: No
USCE Requirement: None
Cut-Off time since graduation: 4 years
Program offers couple match: Yes
Visas Sponsored or accepted: J1 visa and H1b visa

Albert Einstein Healthcare Network Emergency Medicine Residency Program

Specialty: Emergency Medicine
Program name: Albert Einstein Healthcare Network Program
Program code: 110-41-21-122
NRMP Code: 1631110C0
Program type: Community-based university affiliated hospital
State: Pennsylvania
Address: Albert Einstein Medical Center
          5501 Old York Rd, Philadelphia, PA 19141
Phone: (215) 456-6336

Fax: (215) 456-6601
Percentage of IMGs in the program: 5%
Minimum USMLE Step 1 Score Requirement:
No limits set
Minimum USMLE Step 2 Score Requirement:
No limits set
Attempts on any step: No limits set
CS required at time of application: Yes
including ECFMG certificate
USCE Requirement: None
Cut-Off time since graduation: No limits set
Program offers couple match: Yes
Visas Sponsored or accepted: J1 visa and H1b
visa

York Hospital Emergency Medicine Residency Program

Specialty: Emergency Medicine
Program name: York Hospital Program
Program code: 110-41-21-089
NRMP Code: 1674110C0
Program type: Community-based University
affiliated hospital
State: Pennsylvania
Address: York Hospital
         1001 S George St, York, PA 17405
Phone: (717) 851-5064

Fax: (717) 851-3469
Percentage of IMGs in the program: 10%
Minimum USMLE Step 1 Score Requirement: No limits set
Minimum USMLE Step 2 Score Requirement: No limits set
Attempts on any step: No limits set
CS required at time of application: No
USCE Requirement: Yes including two SLOR
Cut-Off time since graduation: No limits set
Program offers couple match: Yes
Visas Sponsored or accepted: J1 visa and H1b visa

Thomas Jefferson University Emergency Medicine Residency Program

Specialty: Emergency Medicine
Program name: Thomas Jefferson University Program
Program code: 110-41-12-064
NRMP Code: 1630110C0
Program type: University-based
State: Pennsylvania
Address: Thomas Jefferson University Hospital
1020 Sansom St, Philadelphia, PA 19107
Phone: (215) 955-9837

Fax: (215) 955-9870
Percentage of IMGs in the program: 10%
Minimum USMLE Step 1 Score Requirement:
No limits set
Minimum USMLE Step 2 Score Requirement:
No limits set
Attempts on any step: No limits set
CS required at time of application: No
USCE Requirement: None
Cut-Off time since graduation: No limits set
Program offers couple match: Yes
Visas Sponsored or accepted: J1 visa and H1b
visa

Texas

Baylor College of Medicine Emergency Medicine Residency Program

Specialty: Emergency Medicine
Program name: Baylor College of Medicine
Program
Program code: 110-48-21-207
State: Texas
Address: Baylor College of Medicine
            1504 Taub Loop, Houston, TX 77030
Phone: (713) 873-2626

Fax: (713) 873-2325
Percentage of IMGs in the program: 10%
Minimum USMLE Step 1 Score Requirement:
No limits set
Minimum USMLE Step 2 Score Requirement:
No limits set
Attempts on any step: No limits set
CS required at time of application: No
USCE Requirement: None
Cut-Off time since graduation: No limits set
Program offers couple match: Yes
Visas Sponsored or accepted: J1 visa and H1b
visa

University of Texas at Houston Emergency Medicine Residency Program

Specialty: Emergency Medicine
Program name: University of Texas at Houston
Program
Program code: 110-48-21-096
NRMP Code: 2923110C0
Program type: University-based
State: Texas
Address: University of Texas HSC Houston
          6431 Fannin St, Houston, TX 77030
Phone: (713) 500-5903
Fax: (713) 500-0758

Percentage of IMGs in the program: 0% (occasionally 1)
Minimum USMLE Step 1 Score Requirement: No limits set
Minimum USMLE Step 2 Score Requirement: No limits set
Attempts on any step: Must pass on maximum the 3rd attempt
CS required at time of application: Yes including ECFMG certificate
USCE Requirement: None
Cut-Off time since graduation: No limits set
Program offers couple match: Yes
Visas Sponsored or accepted: J1 visa

John Peter Smith Hospital (Tarrant County Hospital District) Emergency Medicine Residency Program

Specialty: Emergency Medicine
Program name: John Peter Smith Hospital (Tarrant County Hospital District) Program
Program code: 110-48-12-202
State: Texas
Address: John Peter Smith Hospital
1500 S Main St, Fort Worth, TX 76104
Phone: (817) 702-5613
Fax: (817) 702-1143

Percentage of IMGs in the program: 10%
Minimum USMLE Step 1 Score Requirement:
No limits set
Minimum USMLE Step 2 Score Requirement:
No limits set
Attempts on any step: No limits set
CS required at time of application: Yes
including ECFMG certificate
USCE Requirement: None
Cut-Off time since graduation: No limits set
Program offers couple match: Yes
Visas Sponsored or accepted: No visa

University of Texas Southwestern Medical School (Austin) Emergency Medicine Residency Program

Specialty: Emergency Medicine
Program name: University of Texas
Southwestern Medical School (Austin) Program
Program code: 110-48-00-211
State: Texas
Address: University of Texas Southwestern
Medical School Austin
          1400 IH 35 North, Austin, TX 78701
Phone: (512) 324-8221
Fax: (512) 324-8223
Percentage of IMGs in the program: 15%

Minimum USMLE Step 1 Score Requirement:
No limits set
Minimum USMLE Step 2 Score Requirement:
No limits set
Attempts on any step: No limits set
CS required at time of application: No
USCE Requirement: None
Cut-Off time since graduation: No limits set
Program offers couple match: Yes
Visas Sponsored or accepted: J1 visa

Utah

University of Utah Emergency Medicine Residency Program

Specialty: Emergency Medicine
Program name: University of Utah Program
Program code: 110-49-21-178
State: Utah
Address: University of Utah Medical Center
30 N 1900 E, Salt Lake City, UT 84132
Phone: (801) 581-2272
Fax: (801) 585-0603
Percentage of IMGs in the program: 0%
(occasionally one)

Minimum USMLE Step 1 Score Requirement:
No limits set
Minimum USMLE Step 2 Score Requirement:
No limits set
Attempts on any step: No limits set
CS required at time of application: Yes
including ECFMG certificate
USCE Requirement: None
Cut-Off time since graduation: No limits set
Program offers couple match: Yes
Visas Sponsored or accepted: J1 visa

Virginia

Virginia Commonwealth University Health System Emergency Medicine Residency Program

Specialty: Emergency Medicine
Program name: Virginia Commonwealth University Health System Program
Program code: 110-51-21-160
NRMP Code: 1743110C0
Program type: University-based
State: Virginia
Address: Virginia Commonwealth University Health System

1250 E Marshall St, Richmond, VA 23298
Phone: (804) 828-4860
Fax: (804) 828-4603
Percentage of IMGs in the program: 0% (occasionally one)
Minimum USMLE Step 1 Score Requirement: No limits set
Minimum USMLE Step 2 Score Requirement: No limits set
Attempts on any step: No limits set
CS required at time of application: No
USCE Requirement: Yes
Cut-Off time since graduation: No limits set
Program offers couple match: Yes
Visas Sponsored or accepted: J1 visa

Contents

Please take 1 minute to write a review and rate our book on Amazon. We wish you a successful match. Thank you for buying our book.

If you have any questions please email us at applicantguide@yahoo.com

IMG Guide
&
Applicant Guide

www.imgguide.com
www.applicantguide.com